I0416547

POLYCYSTIC KIDNEY DISEASE
COOKBOOK FOR BEGINNERS

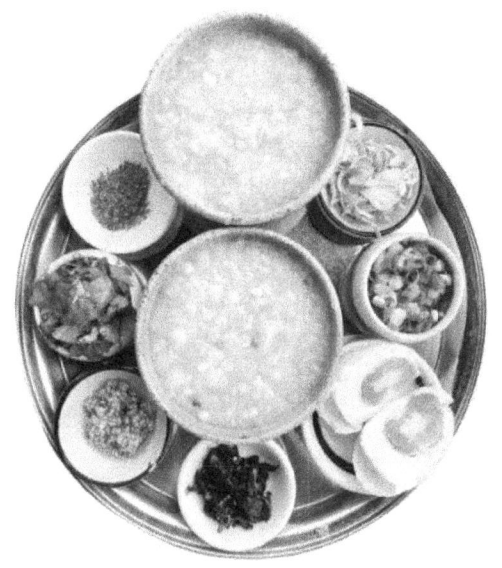

"40 Nutritious Recipes to help Control PKD

for Beginners"

ALLIE NAGEL

DISCLAIMER

This cookbook is intended to provide general information and recipes.

The recipes provided in this cookbook are not intended to replace or be a substitute for medical advice from a physician.

The reader should consult a healthcare professional for any specific medical advice, diagnosis or treatment.

Any specific dietary advice provided in this cookbook is not intended to replace or be a substitute for medical advice from a physician.

The author is not responsible or liable for any adverse effects experienced by readers of this cookbook as a result of following the recipes or dietary advice provided.

The author makes no representations or warranties of any kind (express or implied) as to the accuracy, completeness, reliability or suitability of the recipes provided in this cookbook.

The author disclaims any and all liability for any damages arising out of the use or misuse of the recipes provided in this cookbook. The reader must also take care to ensure that the recipes provided in this cookbook are prepared and cooked safely.

The recipes provided in this cookbook are for informational purposes only and should not be used as a substitute for professional medical advice, diagnosis or treatment.

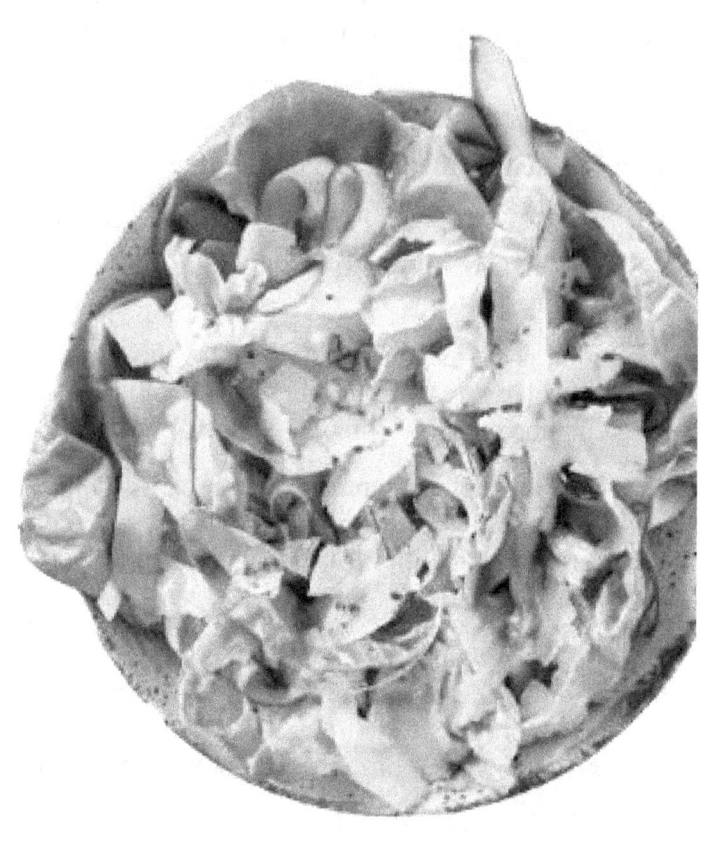

TABLE OF CONTENTS

INTRODUCTION

PKD is a hereditary condition marked by the development of cysts filled with fluid in the kidneys.

It is one of the most common hereditary kidney conditions, impacting individuals of all ages and ethnic backgrounds.

The two primary forms of PKD are Autosomal Dominant Polycystic Kidney Disease (ADPKD) and Autosomal Recessive Polycystic Kidney Disease (ARPKD).

In ADPKD, which is the more prevalent form, an affected individual inherits a mutated gene from one parent. The presence of this mutated gene leads to the development of cysts in both kidneys over time.

These cysts gradually enlarge, causing the kidneys to increase in size and lose their functional capacity. ADPKD symptoms typically manifest in adulthood, and complications may include high blood pressure, kidney stones, and an increased risk of aneurysms.

ARPKD, on the other hand, is a rarer and more severe form of PKD that is usually diagnosed in infancy or childhood. For a child to be affected, both parents need to possess a copy of the mutated gene. In ARPKD, cysts form not only in the kidneys but also in other organs, such as the liver and lungs. This can result in severe complications, including respiratory and hepatic issues.

Common symptoms of PKD include pain or tenderness in the abdomen, frequent urination, blood in the urine, and high blood pressure. Diagnosis often involves imaging tests such as ultrasound, CT scans, or MRI to visualize the cysts within the kidneys.

While there is no cure for PKD, management focuses on alleviating symptoms, slowing the progression of kidney damage, and addressing associated complications.

Lifestyle modifications, including a low-sodium diet, blood pressure control, and staying adequately hydrated, can help manage the condition. In some cases, medical interventions such as pain management and surgery may be necessary.

Regular monitoring and early intervention are crucial for individuals with PKD to maintain kidney function and overall health.

CHAPTER 1

HOW DIET INFLUENCES PKD MANAGEMENT

1. **Blood Pressure Control:** High blood pressure is a common complication of PKD and can accelerate kidney damage. A diet low in sodium helps manage blood pressure. Limiting processed foods, canned goods, and restaurant meals can help reduce sodium intake.

2. **Fluid Balance:** Maintaining proper fluid balance is crucial for you with PKD. Adequate hydration supports overall kidney health, while excessive fluid intake can contribute to cyst growth. Monitoring fluid intake and adjusting it based on individual needs is important.

3. **Protein Intake:** Moderate protein intake is recommended for individuals with PKD. While protein is essential for overall health, excessive protein consumption may increase the kidneys' workload. Choosing high-quality protein sources and moderating portion sizes is advised.

4. **Phosphorus and Calcium Balance:** PKD can affect the balance of phosphorus and calcium in the body. Foods high in phosphorus, such as dairy products and certain nuts, may need to be limited. Adequate calcium intake is important for bone health, and adjustments may be needed based on individual needs.

5. **Glycemic Control:** For you with diabetes and PKD, maintaining stable blood sugar levels is crucial. Choosing complex carbohydrates with a low Glycemic Index helps regulate blood sugar, reducing the risk of complications associated with diabetes.

6. **Omega-3 Fatty Acids:** Including sources of omega-3 fatty acids in the diet, such as fatty fish (e.g., salmon) or flaxseeds, may have anti-inflammatory effects and benefit kidney health.

7. **Limiting Caffeine and Alcohol:** Caffeine and alcohol can affect blood pressure and hydration levels. Moderation or avoidance may be recommended, depending on individual health status.

8. **Weight Management:** Maintaining a healthy weight through a balanced diet and regular exercise is important for overall well-being. Excess weight can contribute to hypertension and other complications associated with PKD.

9. **Phytochemical-Rich Foods:** Consuming fruits and vegetables rich in phytochemicals may have antioxidant and anti-inflammatory effects, potentially benefiting kidney health.

10. **Vitamin D Supplementation:** Vitamin D levels may be affected in PKD, and supplementation may be necessary. Dietary sources of vitamin D include fortified foods like milk and fatty fish.

THE IMPORTANCE OF EARLY DIETARY CHANGES

1. **Blood Pressure Management:** Early dietary changes can help control blood pressure, a critical factor in slowing the progression of kidney damage associated with PKD.

2. **Preventing Fluid Overload:** Monitoring and adjusting fluid intake early on can prevent fluid

overload, reducing the risk of complications such as swelling and high blood pressure.

3. **Reducing Cyst Growth:** Certain dietary modifications may help regulate the growth of kidney cysts, potentially slowing their development.

4. **Minimizing Protein Load:** Early adjustments to protein intake can help minimize the workload on the kidneys, supporting overall kidney function.

5. **Balancing Phosphorus and Calcium:** Managing phosphorus and calcium levels through dietary changes can help maintain a healthy balance, promoting bone health and preventing complications.

6. **Preventing Electrolyte Imbalances:** Early dietary measures can prevent imbalances in electrolytes, which are crucial for proper kidney function.

7. **Blood Sugar Control (for PKD with Diabetes):** Individuals with PKD and diabetes can benefit from early dietary changes to control blood sugar levels and minimize the impact on kidney health.

8. **Maintaining Healthy Weight:** Early dietary interventions can contribute to weight management,

reducing the risk of complications associated with excess weight.

9. **Optimizing Vitamin and Mineral Intake:** Ensuring adequate intake of essential vitamins and minerals through dietary changes supports overall health and compensates for potential deficiencies.

10. **Reducing Oxidative Stress:** Antioxidant-rich foods can be incorporated early on to help reduce oxidative stress and inflammation associated with PKD.

11. **Promoting Heart Health:** Heart health is closely linked to kidney health. Early dietary changes can support cardiovascular well-being, reducing the risk of related complications.

12. **Modulating Sodium Intake:** Limiting sodium intake early in the course of PKD can help manage blood pressure and reduce the risk of fluid retention.

13. **Alleviating Symptoms:** Early dietary modifications can help alleviate symptoms such as abdominal pain, discomfort, and bloating associated with PKD.

14. **Enhancing Immune Function:** A well-balanced diet early on can enhance immune function,

promoting overall health and aiding in the prevention of infections.

15. **Improving Quality of Life:** Early dietary changes contribute to an improved quality of life for individuals with PKD by minimizing symptoms, reducing complications, and supporting overall well-being.

FOODS TO LIMIT OR AVOID FOR PKD MANAGEMENT

1. **Processed Foods:** Processed foods often contain high levels of sodium, which can contribute to high blood pressure and fluid retention. Limiting processed foods helps manage these issues.

2. **Canned Goods:** Canned goods are typically high in sodium. Reducing canned food intake helps control sodium levels, supporting blood pressure management.

3. **Fast Food:** Fast food is often loaded with salt and unhealthy fats, contributing to high blood pressure and cardiovascular issues. Limiting fast food is crucial for overall kidney health.

4. **Sugary Beverages:** Sugary drinks can contribute to weight gain and blood sugar fluctuations. Individuals with PKD, especially those with diabetes, should limit or avoid sugary beverages.

5. **Red Meat:** Red meat is high in protein and can contribute to an increased workload on the kidneys. Moderation or substitution with lean protein sources is recommended.

6. **High-Phosphorus Foods:** Foods high in phosphorus, such as dairy products, nuts, and seeds, may need to be limited as PKD can affect phosphorus balance.

7. **High-Potassium Foods:** Some fruits (e.g., bananas, oranges) and vegetables (e.g., potatoes, tomatoes) are high in potassium. Individuals with PKD and compromised kidney function may need to limit these foods.

8. **Whole Wheat Bread:** While whole wheat is generally a healthy choice, individuals with PKD may need to limit whole wheat bread due to its higher phosphorus content.

9. **Dark Cola:** Dark colas contain phosphoric acid, which may contribute to phosphorus imbalance. Choosing light-colored sodas or, better yet, water is recommended.

10. **Alcohol:** Excessive alcohol consumption can impact blood pressure and contribute to dehydration. Limiting alcohol intake is crucial for individuals with PKD.

11. **Salty Snacks:** Snacks like chips and pretzels are high in sodium. Opting for low-sodium alternatives helps control salt intake.

12. **Caffeine:** Caffeine can raise blood pressure and may contribute to dehydration. Moderation or choosing decaffeinated options is advised.

13. **Deli Meats:** Deli meats are often high in sodium and preservatives. Choosing fresh, lean meats is a healthier alternative.

14. **Pickled Foods:** Pickled foods, such as pickles and olives, are high in sodium. Reducing their intake supports overall sodium control.

15. **High-Sugar Foods:** High-sugar foods can contribute to weight gain and blood sugar fluctuations. Limiting

sugary treats helps manage these factors, especially for those with diabetes.

SAFE AND EFFECTIVE EXERCISES FOR PKD PATIENTS

1. **Walking:** Walking is a low-impact exercise that is gentle on the joints and cardiovascular system. It helps improve overall fitness without putting excessive strain on the kidneys.

2. **Cycling:** Cycling, whether stationary or on a bike, is a great cardiovascular exercise that is gentle on the joints. It promotes cardiovascular health without impacting the kidneys.

3. **Swimming:** Swimming is a form of low-impact exercise that offers a comprehensive workout for the entire body. It is easy on the joints and is generally considered safe for individuals with PKD.

4. **Yoga:** Yoga promotes flexibility, strength, and relaxation. Gentle yoga poses can be adapted to individual fitness levels and are generally safe for PKD patients.

5. **Pilates:** Pilates focuses on core strength, flexibility, and overall muscle toning. Modified Pilates exercises can be beneficial for individuals with PKD.

6. **Tai Chi:** Tai Chi is a low-impact exercise that emphasizes slow, controlled movements. It promotes balance, flexibility, and relaxation.

7. **Stationary Cycling:** Using a stationary bike is an excellent cardiovascular exercise without the impact on the joints. It allows for customizable intensity levels.

8. **Resistance Training with Light Weights:** Incorporating light weights into resistance training helps build muscle strength. However, it's essential to start with low resistance and progress gradually.

9. **Elliptical Training:** The elliptical machine provides a low-impact, full-body workout. It's gentle on the joints and can be adjusted to different intensity levels.

10. **Seated Exercises:** For individuals with mobility challenges, seated exercises can be effective. Seated leg lifts, arm circles, and seated marches are examples.

11. **Gentle Aerobics:** Low-impact aerobic exercises, such as modified aerobics or low-impact dance, can improve cardiovascular health without putting stress on the kidneys.

12. **Rowing Machine:** Rowing provides a full-body workout with minimal impact. It engages various muscle groups and is a safe option for PKD patients.

13. **Stretching:** Incorporating regular stretching exercises helps maintain flexibility and prevents muscle stiffness. It is a safe and beneficial addition to any exercise routine.

14. **Balance Exercises:** Balance exercises, such as standing on one leg or heel-to-toe walking, can help improve stability and prevent falls.

15. **Mindful Breathing Exercises:** Mindful breathing exercises, such as diaphragmatic breathing or deep breathing, promote relaxation and can be incorporated into any exercise routine.

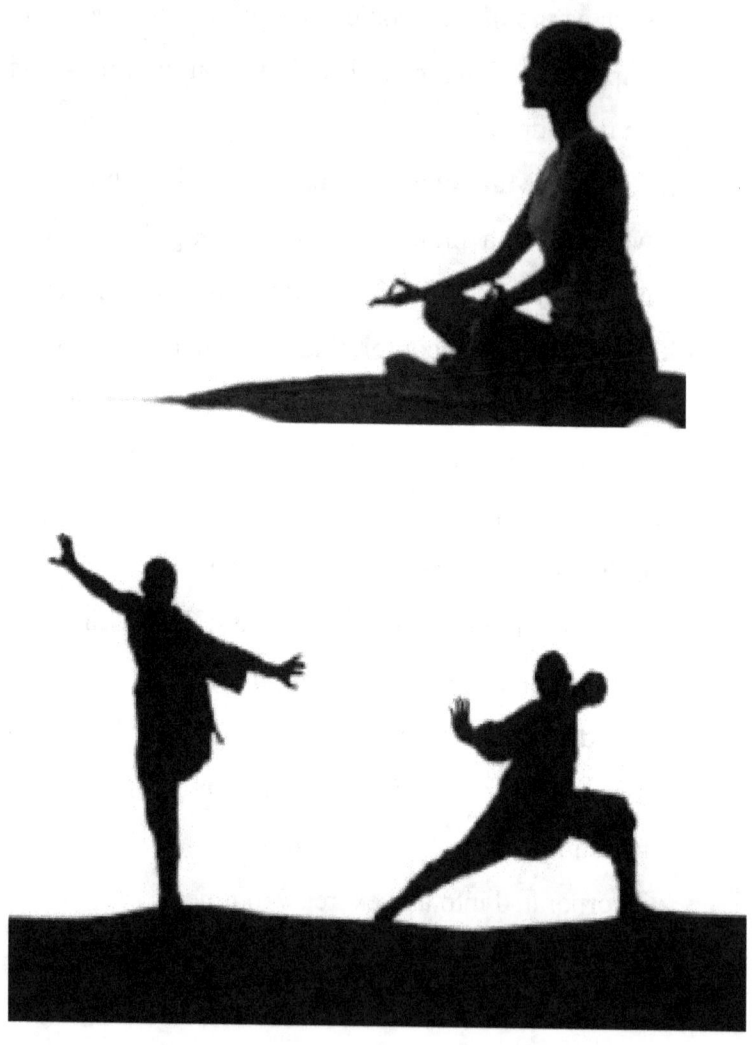

CHAPTER 2

14-DAY MEAL PLAN

DAY 1

Breakfast: Melon and Lettuce Salad

Lunch: Grilled Chicken Salad with Cabbage Sauce

Dinner: Grilled Turkey Burgers with Lettuce Wraps

DAY 2

Breakfast: Wild Rice Porridge with Strawberries

Lunch: Chicken Lettuce Salad

Dinner: Baked Salmon with Dill, served with Asparagus

DAY 3

Breakfast: Peach Smoothie with Macadamia Milk

Lunch: Vegetable Soup with Lettuce and Bell Peppers

Dinner: Vegetable Stew with Carrots, Green Beans, and Celery

DAY 4

Breakfast: Vegetable Omelet with Lettuce

Lunch: Smoked Salmon Salad on Whole Wheat Bread

Dinner: Grilled Chicken Lettuce Salad

DAY 5

Breakfast: Vegetable Omelet with Egg Whites

Lunch: Beef Stew with Carrots and Celery

Dinner: Herb Chicken with Lettuce and Bell Peppers

DAY 6

Breakfast: Eggplant Parmesan with No-Sodium

Lunch: Baked Cod with Herbs

Dinner: Chicken and Rice Casserole with Peas and Carrots

DAY 7

Breakfast: Wild Rice Pudding

Lunch: Shrimp and Broccoli Stir-Fry

Dinner: Grilled Shrimp Salad with Mixed Greens and Vinaigrette

DAY 8

Breakfast: Egg White Salad with Whole White Bread Sandwich

Lunch: Whole Wheat Pasta with Garlic and Olive Oil

Dinner: Baked Cod with Pepper Seasoning and Sautéed Lettuce

DAY 9

Breakfast: White Bread French Toast with Applesauce

Lunch: Fresh Turkey Burger

Dinner: Baked Tilapia with Steamed Kale

DAY 10

Breakfast: Rice Cake with Apple and Cinnamon

Lunch: Cauliflower Salad with Peas and Carrots

Dinner: Cauliflower Rice Stir-Fry with Mixed Vegetables

DAY 11

Breakfast: Melon and Lettuce Salad

Lunch: Grilled Chicken Salad with Cabbage Sauce

Dinner: Grilled Turkey Burgers with Lettuce Wraps

DAY 12

Breakfast: Wild Rice Porridge with Strawberries

Lunch: Chicken Lettuce Salad

Dinner: Baked Salmon with Dill, served with Asparagus

DAY 13

Breakfast: Peach Smoothie with Macadamia Milk

Lunch: Vegetable Soup with Lettuce and Bell Peppers

Dinner: Vegetable Stew with Carrots, Green Beans, and Celery

DAY 14

Breakfast: Vegetable Omelet with Lettuce

Lunch: Smoked Salmon Salad on Whole Wheat Bread

Dinner: Grilled Chicken Lettuce Salad

CHAPTER 3

40 NUTRITIOUS RECIPES FOR A PKD DIET

BREAKFAST

Melon and Lettuce Salad

Preparation Time: 15 minutes

Serves: 4

Calories: 120 **Sodium:** 10mg **Sugar:** 0g

Ingredients:

2 cups chopped romaine lettuce

1 cup diced cantaloupe

1 cup diced honeydew melon

Bell pepper

1/4 cup sliced cucumber

2 tablespoons olive oil

1 tablespoon balsamic vinegar

Pepper

Method of Preparation:

1. In a large bowl, combine romaine lettuce, cantaloupe, honeydew melon, bell pepper, and cucumber.
2. In a small bowl, whisk together olive oil and balsamic vinegar.
3. Pour over the salad.
4. Toss the salad until evenly coated.
5. Season with Pepper.
6. Serve immediately.

Wild Rice Porridge with Strawberries

Preparation Time: 25 minutes

Serves: 2

Calories: 250 **Sodium:** 20mg **Sugar:** 8g

Ingredients:

1 cup wild rice (low in potassium, phosphorus, sodium)

2 cups water

1 cup almond milk (low in phosphorus, saturated fat)

1/2 cup blueberries

1 tablespoon honey (optional)

1/4 teaspoon cinnamon

1/4 teaspoon vanilla extract

Method of Preparation:

1. Rinse rice under cold water.
2. In a pot, combine rice and water.
3. Bring to a boil, then reduce heat and simmer until rice is tender.
4. Add almond milk, strawberries, honey (if using), cinnamon, and vanilla extract. Stir well.
5. Simmer for an additional 5-7 minutes, until blueberries are soft and flavors are well combined.
6. Remove from heat, let it cool slightly, and serve.

Peach Smoothie with Macadamia Milk

Preparation Time: 10 minutes

Serves: 1

Calories: 220 **Sodium:** 40mg **Sugar:** 3g

Ingredients:

1 cup frozen peaches (low in potassium, phosphorus, sodium)

1/2 cup macadamia milk

1 tablespoon chia seeds

1 teaspoon honey (optional)

Ice cubes (optional)

Method of Preparation:

1. In a blender, combine frozen peaches, macadamia milk, chia seeds, and honey (if using).
2. Blend until smooth and creamy.
3. Add ice cubes if a colder consistency is desired, then blend again.

4. Pour into a glass and serve.

Vegetable Omelet with Lettuce

Preparation Time: 15 minutes

Serves: 1

Calories: 280 **Sodium:** 280mg **Sugar:** 3g

Ingredients:

2 eggs

1/4 cup diced bell peppers

1/4 cup spinach (low in potassium, phosphorus, sodium)

1 tablespoon olive oil

Pepper

1 cup shredded lettuce

Method of Preparation:

1. In a bowl, beat eggs and season with pepper.
2. Heat olive oil in a non-stick skillet over medium heat.
3. Add bell peppers, and spinach to the skillet. Sauté until vegetables are tender.

4. Pour beaten eggs over the vegetables, swirling to spread evenly.

5. Cook until the edges are set, then flip and cook the other side until eggs are fully cooked.

6. Slide the omelet onto a plate, serve with shredded lettuce on the side.

Vegetable Omelet with Egg Whites

Preparation Time: 15 minutes

Serves: 2

Calories: 120 **Sodium:** 150mg **Sugar:** 2g

Ingredients:

6 egg whites

1/2 cup diced bell peppers

1/4 cup chopped spinach

1/4 cup diced onions

1/4 teaspoon black pepper

1/4 teaspoon low-sodium seasoning

1 teaspoon olive oil (low-sodium)

Method of Preparation:

1. In a bowl, whisk together the egg whites, black pepper, and low-sodium seasoning.
2. Heat olive oil in a non-stick skillet over medium heat.
3. Add onions, and bell peppers to the skillet. Sauté until softened.
4. Pour the egg white mixture over the vegetables.
5. Allow it to cook, lifting the edges to let uncooked egg flow underneath.
6. Once the omelet is set, fold it in half and serve.

Eggplant Parmesan with No-Sodium

Preparation Time: 45 minutes

Serves: 4

Calories: 280 **Sodium:** 120mg **Sugar:** 6g

Ingredients:

1 large eggplant, sliced

Bell pepper

1 cup shredded low-fat mozzarella cheese

1/2 cup grated Parmesan cheese

1/2 cup whole-grain breadcrumbs

1 teaspoon dried oregano

1 teaspoon dried basil

1/2 teaspoon garlic powder

Method of Preparation:

1. Preheat oven to 375°F (190°C).
2. Dip eggplant slices in beaten egg, then coat with breadcrumbs.
3. Arrange slices on a baking sheet and bake until golden brown.
4. In a separate bowl, bell pepper sauce, oregano, basil, and garlic powder.
5. In a baking dish, layer eggplant, bell pepper sauce, and cheeses. Repeat.
6. Bake until cheese is melted and bubbly.

Wild Rice Pudding

Preparation Time: 30 minutes

Serves: 3

Calories: 180 **Sodium:** 80mg **Sugar:** 10g

Ingredients:

1 cup cooked wild rice

2 cups unsweetened almond milk (low-sodium)

1/4 cup honey or maple syrup

1/2 teaspoon vanilla extract

1/2 teaspoon ground cinnamon

1/4 cup chopped almonds (optional)

Method of Preparation:

1. In a saucepan, combine cooked wild rice, almond milk, honey (or maple syrup), vanilla extract, and cinnamon.
2. Bring to a simmer and cook, stirring frequently, until thickened.
3. Remove from heat and let it cool.
4. Optionally, top with chopped almonds before Serves.

Egg White Salad with Whole White Bread Sandwich

Preparation Time: 20 minutes

Serves: 4

Calories: 250 **Sodium:** 300mg **Sugar:** 1g

Ingredients:

6 large egg whites

1/4 cup low-fat mayonnaise

2 teaspoons Dijon mustard

1/4 cup finely chopped celery

2 tablespoons finely chopped green onions

Pepper

8 slices whole white bread (low-sodium)

Method of Preparation:

1. Hard boil the egg whites, then chop them.
2. In a bowl, mix chopped egg whites, mayonnaise, Dijon mustard, celery, green onions, and pepper.

3. Spread the egg white salad onto 4 slices of whole white bread and top with the remaining slices to form sandwiches.

White Bread French Toast with Applesauce

Preparation Time: 15 minutes

Serves: 2

Calories: 220 **Sodium:** 200mg **Sugar:** 5g

Ingredients:

4 slices white bread (low-sodium)

1 cup egg substitute

1/2 cup skim milk

1 teaspoon vanilla extract

1/2 teaspoon ground cinnamon

Cooking spray

1 cup unsweetened applesauce

Method of Preparation:

1. In a bowl, whisk together egg substitute, skim milk, vanilla extract, and cinnamon.

2. Dip each slice of white bread into the mixture, ensuring both sides are coated.

3. Cook on a griddle or skillet sprayed with cooking spray until golden brown on both sides.

4. Serve with a side of unsweetened applesauce.

Rice Cake with Apple and Cinnamon

Preparation Time: 10 minutes

Serves: 2

Calories: 120 **Sodium:** 5mg **Sugar:** 8g

Ingredients:

2 rice cakes (low-sodium and low-phosphorus)

1 medium apple, thinly sliced (choose a low-potassium variety, like Granny Smith)

1/2 teaspoon ground cinnamon

1 teaspoon honey (optional, adjust based on personal preference)

Method of Preparation:

Wash and thinly slice the apple.

1. If following a low-potassium diet, choose varieties that are lower in potassium, such as Granny Smith apples.
2. Choose low-sodium and low-phosphorus rice cakes. Toast them to your liking.
3. Place the sliced apples on top of the rice cakes.
4. Sprinkle ground cinnamon over the apple slices.
5. Drizzle with Maple syrup if desired.
6. Adjust the amount based on your taste preferences.

LUNCH

Grilled Chicken Salad with Cabbage Sauce

Preparation Time: 25 minutes

Serves: 4

Calories: 320 **Sodium:** 120mg **Sugar:** 5g

Ingredients:

1 lb. boneless, skinless chicken breasts

1 small green cabbage, shredded

2 carrots, julienned

Bell pepper

1 cucumber, sliced

1/4 cup olive oil

2 tablespoons apple cider vinegar

1 teaspoon Dijon mustard

Pepper

Method of Preparation:

1. Season chicken breasts with pepper, then grill until fully cooked.
2. In a bowl, mix shredded cabbage, julienned carrots, bell pepper, and cucumber.
3. Slice grilled chicken and place on top of the vegetable mix.

4. In a separate bowl, whisk together olive oil, apple cider vinegar, Dijon mustard, and pepper to create the cabbage sauce.

5. Drizzle the cabbage sauce over the salad before Serves.

Chicken Lettuce Salad

Preparation Time: 20 minutes

Serves: 3

Calories: 280 **Sodium:** 180mg **Sugar:** 6g

Ingredients:

1 lb. grilled chicken breast, sliced

1 head of lettuce, torn

Bell pepper

1/2 red onion, thinly sliced

1/4 cup balsamic vinaigrette dressing

1/4 cup feta cheese, crumbled (optional)

Pepper

Method of Preparation:

1. Combine torn lettuce, bell pepper, and sliced red onion in a large bowl.
2. Top with grilled chicken slices.
3. Drizzle balsamic vinaigrette over the salad and toss gently.
4. Sprinkle with crumbled feta cheese if desired.
5. Season with Pepper.

Vegetable Soup with Lettuce and Bell Peppers

Preparation Time: 30 minutes

Serves: 5

Calories: 120 **Sodium:** 150mg **Sugar:** 4g

Ingredients:

2 cups lettuce, chopped

1 red bell pepper, diced

1 yellow bell pepper, diced

1 zucchini, sliced

1 cup carrots, chopped

4 cups low-sodium vegetable broth

1 teaspoon olive oil

1 teaspoon dried thyme

Pepper

Method of Preparation:

1. In a pot, sauté bell peppers, zucchini, and carrots in olive oil until slightly tender.
2. Add lettuce and continue to sauté for a few minutes.
3. Pour in the vegetable broth, add dried thyme and pepper.
4. Bring to a simmer and let it cook until vegetables are fully cooked.

Smoked Salmon Salad on Whole Wheat Bread

Preparation Time: 15 minutes

Serves: 4

Calories: 300 **Sodium:** 250mg **Sugar:** 2g

Ingredients:

8 oz smoked salmon (low-sodium)

4 slices of low-phosphorus, whole wheat bread

2 cups mixed salad greens (kale, spinach, arugula)

Bell pepper

1/2 cucumber, sliced

1/4 red onion, thinly sliced

2 tbsp olive oil

1 tbsp balsamic vinegar

Pepper

Method of Preparation:

1. In a large bowl, combine salad greens, bell pepper, cucumber, and red onion.
2. Drizzle olive oil and balsamic vinegar over the salad, toss gently.
3. Place smoked salmon on whole wheat bread slices.
4. Serve the smoked salmon on bread alongside the salad.

Beef Stew with Carrots and Celery

Preparation Time: 30 Minutes

Serves: 6

Calories: 320 **Sodium:** 200mg **Sugar:** 3g

Ingredients:

1.5 lb. lean beef stew meat, cubed

4 carrots, peeled and sliced

4 celery stalks, chopped

1 onion, diced

3 cloves garlic, minced

4 cups low-sodium beef broth

Bell pepper

1 tsp thyme

1 tsp rosemary

Pepper

Method of Preparation:

1. In a large pot, brown beef over medium heat.
2. Add onion and garlic, cook until softened.
3. Stir in carrots, celery, beef broth, blended bell pepper, thyme, rosemary, and pepper.
4. Simmer for 1.5-2 hours until meat is tender.

Baked Cod with Herbs

Preparation Time: 25 minutes

Serves: 4

Calories: 200 **Sodium:** 150mg **Sugar:** 0g

Ingredients:

4 cod fillets

2 tbsp olive oil

2 tbsp fresh lemon juice

2 tsp dried oregano

1 tsp dried thyme

1 tsp garlic powder

Pepper

Method of Preparation:

1. Preheat oven to 375°F (190°C).
2. Place cod fillets in a baking dish.
3. Mix olive oil, lemon juice, oregano, thyme, garlic powder and pepper.
4. Drizzle mixture over cod, ensuring it's well-coated.
5. Bake for 15-20 minutes or until fish flakes easily.

Shrimp and Broccoli Stir-Fry

Preparation Time: 25 minutes

Serves: 4

Calories: 350 **Sodium:** 450mg **Sugar:** 3g

Ingredients:

1 lb. shrimp, peeled and deveined

2 cups broccoli florets

1 red bell pepper, sliced

2 cloves garlic, minced

1 tablespoon ginger, grated

3 tablespoons low-sodium soy sauce

1 tablespoon oyster sauce

1 tablespoon sesame oil

1 tablespoon canola oil

2 green onions, chopped

2 cups cooked brown rice

Method of Preparation:

1. In a wok or large skillet, heat canola oil over medium-high heat.
2. Add shrimp and stir-fry until pink and opaque. Remove shrimp and set aside.
3. In the same pan, add garlic and ginger. Stir-fry for 1 minute.
4. Add broccoli and bell pepper, stir-frying until vegetables are tender-crisp.
5. Return the cooked shrimp to the pan.
6. In a small bowl, mix soy sauce, oyster sauce, and sesame oil. Pour over the shrimp and vegetables.
7. Stir-fry for an additional 2 minutes until everything is well-coated and heated through.

8. Sprinkle with green onions and serve over cooked brown rice.

Whole Wheat Pasta with Garlic and Olive Oil

Preparation Time: 20 minutes

Serves: 4

Calories: 300 **Sodium:** 200mg **Sugar:** 2g

Ingredients:

8 oz whole wheat spaghetti

3 tablespoons olive oil

4 cloves garlic, thinly sliced

1/2 teaspoon red pepper flakes (optional)

Pepper

2 tablespoons fresh parsley, chopped

1/4 cup grated Parmesan cheese (optional)

Method of Preparation:

1. Cook the whole wheat spaghetti according to package instructions.
2. Drain and set aside.
3. In a large pan, heat olive oil over medium heat.
4. Add sliced garlic and red pepper flakes, sautéing until garlic is golden but not burnt.
5. Add the cooked pasta to the pan, tossing to coat evenly with the garlic-infused oil.
6. Season with black pepper to taste.
7. Toss in fresh parsley.
8. Optional: Sprinkle with grated Parmesan cheese before Serves.

Fresh Turkey Burger

Preparation Time: 20 minutes

Serves: 4

Calories: 250 **Sodium:** 200 mg **Sugar:** 1g

Ingredients:

1-pound fresh ground turkey (lean)

1/4 cup finely chopped onion

2 cloves garlic, minced

1 tablespoon Worcestershire sauce

1 teaspoon Dijon mustard

Pepper

Whole-grain burger buns

Lettuce leaves

Method of Preparation:

1. In a mixing bowl, combine ground turkey, chopped onion, minced garlic, Worcestershire sauce, Dijon mustard, and pepper.
2. Mix the ingredients well and form the mixture into burger patties.
3. Grill the turkey burgers over medium heat until fully cooked, approximately 4-5 minutes per side.
4. Toast the whole-grain burger buns on the grill or in a toaster.
5. Assemble the burgers with lettuce leaves and any other preferred toppings.

Cauliflower Salad with Peas and Carrots

Preparation Time: 15 minutes (plus chilling time)

Serves: 6

Calories: 120 **Sodium:** 60 mg **Sugar:** 4g

Ingredients:

1 medium head cauliflower, cut into florets

1 cup frozen peas, thawed

1 cup carrots, finely chopped

1/4 cup red onion, finely chopped

1/4 cup fresh parsley, chopped

1/4 cup olive oil

2 tablespoons apple cider vinegar

Pepper

Method of Preparation:

1. Steam or blanch cauliflower florets until tender-crisp.

2. Allow them to cool.

3. In a large bowl, combine cauliflower, thawed peas, chopped carrots, red onion, and fresh parsley.

4. In a small bowl, whisk together olive oil, apple cider vinegar, and pepper to create the dressing.

5. Pour the dressing over the vegetables and toss gently to coat.

6. Refrigerate the salad for at least 30 minutes before serving.

DINNER

Grilled Turkey Burgers with Lettuce Wraps

Preparation Time: 20 minutes

Serves: 4

Calories: 220 **Sodium:** 120mg **Sugar:** 1g

Ingredients:

1 pound ground turkey (low-fat)

1/2 cup finely chopped onions

2 cloves garlic, minced

1 teaspoon dried oregano

1 teaspoon dried thyme

Pepper

Butter lettuce leaves for wraps

Bell pepper

Method of Preparation:

1. In a bowl, mix ground turkey, onions, garlic, oregano, thyme and pepper.
2. Form the mixture into burger patties.
3. Preheat the grill and cook patties for 5-7 minutes per side or until fully cooked.
4. Serve the turkey burgers in butter lettuce wraps.

Baked Salmon with Dill, served with Asparagus

Preparation Time: 25 minutes

Serves: 4

Calories: 280 **Sodium:** 80mg **Sugar:** 2g

Ingredients:

4 salmon fillets

1 tablespoon olive oil

1 tablespoon fresh dill, chopped

Pepper

1 bunch asparagus, trimmed

Method of Preparation:

1. Preheat the oven to 375°F (190°C).
2. Place salmon fillets on a baking sheet, drizzle with olive oil, sprinkle with dill, and pepper.
3. Arrange asparagus around the salmon.
4. Bake for 15-20 minutes or until salmon is cooked through and flakes easily.

Vegetable Stew with Carrots, Green Beans, and Celery

Preparation Time: 30 minutes

Serves: 6

Calories: 120 **Sodium:** 70mg **Sugar:** 5g

Ingredients:

2 cups carrots, sliced

2 cups green beans, chopped

2 cups celery, diced

1 onion, finely chopped

2 cloves garlic, minced

4 cups low-sodium vegetable broth

1 teaspoon dried thyme

Pepper

Method of Preparation:

1. In a pot, sauté onions and garlic until translucent.
2. Add carrots, green beans, celery, thyme, and pepper.
3. Pour in vegetable broth, bring to a boil, then reduce heat and simmer until vegetables are tender.

Grilled Chicken Lettuce Salad

Preparation Time: 20 minutes

Serves: 4

Calories: 250 **Sodium:** 150mg **Sugar:** 5g

Ingredients:

2 boneless, skinless chicken breasts

1 head of lettuce (choose low potassium varieties like iceberg)

Bell pepper

1 cucumber, sliced

1/4 cup red onion, thinly sliced

2 tablespoons olive oil

2 tablespoons balsamic vinegar

Pepper

Method of Preparation:

1. Season chicken breasts pepper.
2. Grill chicken until fully cooked, approximately 6-8 minutes per side.
3. In a large bowl, combine lettuce, bell pepper, cucumber, and red onion.
4. Slice grilled chicken and place it on top of the salad.

5. In a small bowl, whisk together olive oil and balsamic vinegar.

6. Drizzle over the salad.

7. Toss gently and serve.

Herb Chicken with Lettuce and Bell Peppers

Preparation Time: 40 minutes

Serves: 4

Calories: 280 **Sodium:** 150mg **Sugar:** 2g

Ingredients:

4 boneless, skinless chicken breasts

1 tablespoon olive oil

1 teaspoon dried oregano

1 teaspoon dried thyme

1 teaspoon garlic powder

Pepper

2 cups lettuce, chopped

1 red bell pepper, sliced

1 yellow bell pepper, sliced

Substitutions for Polycystic Kidney Disease (PKD):

Replace regular salt with a low-sodium alternative.

Use herbs and spices for flavor instead of additional salt.

Method of Preparation:

1. Preheat oven to 375°F (190°C).
2. In a small bowl, mix oregano, thyme, garlic powder, and pepper.
3. Rub chicken breasts with olive oil, then sprinkle the herb mixture evenly over both sides.
4. Place chicken breasts in a baking dish and bake for 25-30 minutes or until cooked through.
5. In a large bowl, combine lettuce and sliced bell peppers.
6. Slice cooked chicken and serve over the bed of lettuce and bell peppers.

Chicken and Rice Casserole with Peas and Carrots

Preparation Time: 50 minutes

Serves: 6

Calories: 320 **Sodium:** 180mg **Sugar:** 3g

Ingredients:

1 cup white rice

2 cups cooked chicken, shredded

1 cup frozen peas

1 cup carrots, diced

1 cup low-sodium chicken broth

1 cup low-fat milk

1 tablespoon olive oil

1 teaspoon onion powder

1 teaspoon garlic powder

Pepper

Substitutions for Polycystic Kidney Disease (PKD):

Use low-sodium chicken broth.

Replace regular salt with a low-sodium alternative.

Opt. for low-fat milk.

Method of Preparation:

1. Preheat oven to 350°F (175°C).
2. Cook rice according to package instructions.
3. In a large bowl, combine cooked rice, shredded chicken, frozen peas, and diced carrots.
4. In a separate saucepan, heat olive oil over medium heat. Add onion powder, garlic powder, and pepper.
5. Pour in chicken broth and milk, stirring continuously until the mixture thickens.
6. Pour the sauce over the rice and chicken mixture, stirring to combine.
7. Transfer the mixture to a baking dish and bake for 25-30 minutes or until bubbly.

Grilled Shrimp Salad with Mixed Greens and Vinaigrette

Preparation Time: 20 minutes

Serves: 4

Calories: 320 **Sodium:** 350mg **Sugar:** 3g

Ingredients:

1 pound shrimp, peeled and deveined

8 cups mixed salad greens

Bell pepper

1 cucumber, sliced

1/4 cup red onion, thinly sliced

1/3 cup feta cheese, crumbled (low potassium)

1/4 cup black olives, pitted and sliced (low sodium)

1/4 cup extra-virgin olive oil (EVOO)

2 tablespoons red wine vinegar

1 teaspoon Dijon mustard

Pepper

Method of Preparation:

1. Preheat grill to medium-high heat.
2. Season shrimp with pepper, then grill for 2-3 minutes per side until cooked.
3. In a large bowl, combine mixed greens, bell pepper, cucumber, red onion, feta, and olives.
4. In a small bowl, whisk together EVOO, red wine vinegar, Dijon mustard, and pepper to create the vinaigrette.
5. Toss the salad with grilled shrimp and drizzle the vinaigrette over the top.
6. Serve immediately.

Baked Cod with Pepper Seasoning and Sautéed Lettuce

Preparation Time: 25 minutes

Serves: 4

Calories: 280 **Sodium:** 200mg **Sugar:** 2g

Ingredients:

4 cod fillets (substitute with low phosphorus fish if needed)

1 teaspoon black pepper

1 teaspoon paprika

1 teaspoon garlic powder

1/2 teaspoon onion powder

1/4 teaspoon cayenne pepper (optional)

2 tablespoons olive oil

1 head of lettuce, shredded (substitute with low potassium greens)

Method of Preparation:

1. Preheat oven to 400°F (200°C).
2. In a small bowl, mix black pepper, paprika, garlic powder, onion powder, and cayenne pepper.
3. Place cod fillets on a baking sheet, rub with olive oil, and season with the spice mixture.
4. Bake for 15-20 minutes until the fish is opaque and flakes easily.

5. While the cod is baking, sauté shredded lettuce in a pan with a dash of olive oil until wilted.

6. Serve the baked cod over sautéed lettuce.

Baked Tilapia with Steamed Kale

Preparation Time: 25 minutes

Serves: 4

Calories: 180 **Sodium:** 150mg **Sugar:** 1g

Ingredients:

4 tilapia fillets

1 tablespoon olive oil

1 teaspoon garlic powder

1 teaspoon lemon juice

Pepper

4 cups kale, washed and chopped

Method of Preparation:

1. Preheat the oven to 375°F (190°C).

2. Place tilapia fillets on a baking sheet lined with parchment paper.

3. Drizzle olive oil and lemon juice over the fillets, then sprinkle with garlic powder, and pepper.

4. Bake for 15-20 minutes or until the tilapia is cooked through.

5. While tilapia is baking, steam kale for 5-7 minutes until tender.

6. Serve baked tilapia over steamed kale.

Cauliflower Rice Stir-Fry with Mixed Vegetables

Preparation Time: 20 minutes

Serves: 4

Calories: 120 **Sodium:** 300mg **Sugar:** 4g

Ingredients:

1 head cauliflower, riced

2 tablespoons low-sodium soy sauce

1 tablespoon sesame oil

1 cup broccoli florets

1 cup sliced bell peppers (any color)

1 cup snap peas, trimmed

1 tablespoon olive oil

2 cloves garlic, minced

1 teaspoon grated ginger

Pepper

Method of Preparation:

1. In a large skillet, heat olive oil over medium heat.
2. Add garlic and ginger, sauté for 1-2 minutes.
3. Add broccoli, bell peppers, and snap peas. Stir-fry until vegetables are tender-crisp.
4. Push vegetables to one side of the skillet; add cauliflower rice to the other side.
5. Pour soy sauce and sesame oil over cauliflower rice. Stir-fry for 5-7 minutes until cauliflower is tender.
6. Combine cauliflower rice with vegetables.
7. Season with pepper.

DESSERTS

Baked Apples with Cinnamon

Preparation Time: 15 minutes

Serves: 4

Calories: 150 **Sodium:** 5mg **Sugar:** 15g

Ingredients:

4 large apples, peeled and cored

2 tablespoons cinnamon

2 tablespoons brown sugar (or sugar substitute for a lower sugar option)

1/4 cup chopped walnuts (optional)

1 tablespoon unsalted butter (or low-sodium margarine)

Method of Preparation:

1. Preheat the oven to 375°F (190°C).
2. In a bowl, mix cinnamon, brown sugar, and chopped walnuts.

3. Fill the cored apples with the cinnamon mixture and place them in a baking dish.

4. Top each apple with a small piece of butter.

5. Bake for 25-30 minutes or until apples are tender.

6. Serve warm.

Modified Cheesecake Bites with Almond Flour

Preparation Time: 20 minutes

Serves: 12

Calories: 120 **Sodium:** 30mg **Sugar:** 5g

Ingredients:

2 cups almond flour

1/2 cup low-fat cream cheese

1/4 cup honey (or sugar substitute for a lower sugar option)

2 large eggs

1 teaspoon vanilla extract

Method of Preparation:

1. Preheat the oven to 350°F (175°C).
2. In a bowl, combine almond flour, cream cheese, honey, eggs, and vanilla extract.
3. Mix until well combined.
4. Spoon the mixture into mini muffin cups.
5. Bake for 15-18 minutes or until set.
6. Allow to cool before Serves.

Wild Rice Pudding

Preparation Time: 30 minutes

Serves: 4

Calories: 180 **Sodium:** 20mg **Sugar:** 10g

Ingredients:

1 cup wild rice, cooked

2 cups almond milk (or low-phosphorus milk)

1/4 cup maple syrup (or sugar substitute for a lower sugar option)

1 teaspoon cinnamon

1/4 cup raisins (optional)

Method of Preparation:

1. In a saucepan, combine cooked wild rice and almond milk.
2. Stir in maple syrup and cinnamon.
3. Cook over medium heat until thickened, stirring occasionally.
4. Remove from heat and stir in raisins if desired.
5. Let it cool before Serves.

Strawberry Shortcake

Preparation Time: 45 minutes

Serves: 8

Calories: 350 **Sodium:** 150mg **Sugar:** 15g

Ingredients:

1-pound fresh strawberries, hulled and sliced

1/4 cup granulated sugar

2 cups all-purpose flour

1/4 cup sugar

1 tablespoon baking powder

1/2 cup unsalted butter, cold and cut into small pieces

3/4 cup milk

1 teaspoon vanilla extract

1 cup heavy cream

2 tablespoons powdered sugar

Method of Preparation:

1. In a bowl, combine sliced strawberries with 1/4 cup sugar.
2. Let it sit for 30 minutes to allow the strawberries to release juices.
3. Preheat oven to 425°F (220°C).
4. In a large bowl, whisk together flour, 1/4 cup sugar, and baking powder.
5. Cut in the cold butter until the mixture resembles coarse crumbs.
6. Add milk and vanilla extract to the flour mixture, stirring until just combined.
7. Turn the dough out onto a floured surface and gently knead it a few times.

8. Roll or pat the dough to about 1 inch thickness. Cut out shortcakes using a biscuit cutter.

9. Place the shortcakes on a baking sheet and bake for 12-15 minutes or until golden brown.

10. While the shortcakes cool, whip the heavy cream with powdered sugar until stiff peaks form.

11. To assemble, split the shortcakes in half, spoon strawberries over the bottom half, add a dollop of whipped cream, and top with the other half.

Roasted Pears

Preparation Time: 35 minutes

Serves: 4

Calories: 180 **Sodium:** 5mg **Sugar:** 20g

Ingredients:

4 ripe but firm pears, halved and cored

2 tablespoons honey

1 teaspoon cinnamon

1/4 cup chopped walnuts (optional)

Fresh mint leaves for garnish

Method of Preparation:

1. Preheat the oven to 375°F (190°C).
2. Place pear halves in a baking dish, cut side up.
3. Drizzle honey over the pears and sprinkle with cinnamon. Add chopped walnuts if desired.
4. Roast in the oven for 25-30 minutes or until pears are tender.
5. Garnish with fresh mint leaves before Serves.

STEWS AND SOUPS

Cauliflower Soup with Cod

Preparation Time: 30 minutes

Serves: 4

Calories: 250 **Sodium:** 200mg **Sugar:** 3g

Ingredients:

1 medium cauliflower, chopped

1 pound cod fillets, cut into chunks

1 onion, diced

2 cloves garlic, minced

4 cups low-potassium vegetable broth

1 teaspoon low-sodium seasoning blend

1 tablespoon olive oil (low in saturated fat)

Method of Preparation:

1. In a large pot, sauté onions and garlic in olive oil until softened.
2. Add cauliflower and vegetable broth, bring to a boil, then reduce heat and simmer until cauliflower is tender.
3. Gently add cod chunks and seasoning blend, simmer until cod is cooked through.
4. Serve hot.

Lettuce and Bell Pepper Stew

Preparation Time: 40 minutes

Serves: 6

Calories: 120 **Sodium:** 150mg **Sugar:** 6g

Ingredients:

1 small lettuce, shredded

2 bell peppers, diced

1 onion, chopped

2 cloves garlic, minced

2 cups low-potassium vegetable broth

1 teaspoon olive oil (low in saturated fat)

Method of Preparation:

1. In a large pot, sauté onions and garlic in olive oil until translucent.
2. Add lettuce, bell peppers and vegetable broth.
3. Simmer until vegetables are tender.
4. Season to taste with low-sodium herbs.

Vegetable Broth Soup

Preparation Time: 25 minutes

Serves: 4

Calories: 80 **Sodium:** 100mg **Sugar:** 4g

Ingredients:

4 cups low-potassium vegetable broth

1 cup carrots, sliced

1 cup celery, diced

1 cup zucchini, chopped

1 cup green beans, cut

1 teaspoon olive oil (low in saturated fat)

Herbs and spices to taste (low-sodium)

Method of Preparation:

1. In a pot, sauté carrots, celery, and zucchini in olive oil until slightly softened.
2. Add vegetable broth and bring to a simmer.
3. Add green beans and simmer until all vegetables are tender.
4. Season with low-sodium herbs and spices.

Mushroom Cabbage Soup with Skinless Chicken

Preparation Time: 40 minutes

Serves: 6

Calories: 220 **Sodium:** 300mg **Sugar:** 4g

Ingredients:

1 lb. skinless, boneless chicken breasts, diced

8 cups low-sodium chicken broth

2 cups sliced mushrooms

4 cups shredded green cabbage

1 cup chopped carrots

1 cup diced celery

1 onion, finely chopped

2 cloves garlic, minced

1 teaspoon dried thyme

1 teaspoon dried rosemary

Pepper

2 tablespoons olive oil

Method of Preparation:

1. In a large pot, heat olive oil over medium heat.
2. Add onion and garlic, sauté until softened.

3. Add diced chicken, cook until browned.

4. Pour in chicken broth, add mushrooms, cabbage, carrots, celery, thyme, rosemary, and pepper.

5. Bring to a boil, then reduce heat and simmer for 20-25 minutes until vegetables are tender.

6. Adjust seasoning if needed.

7. Serve hot.

Cabbage and Bell Pepper Soup

Preparation Time: 45 minutes

Serves: 8

Calories: 180 **Sodium:** 250mg **Sugar:** 6g

Ingredients:

1 small cabbage, shredded

2 bell peppers (red and green), diced

1 large onion, finely chopped

3 cloves garlic, minced

8 cups low-sodium vegetable broth

1 teaspoon dried oregano

1 teaspoon dried basil

Pepper

2 tablespoons olive oil

Method of Preparation:

1. Heat olive oil in a large pot.
2. Add onions and garlic, sauté until fragrant.
3. Add bell peppers and cabbage, cook until slightly softened.
4. Pour in vegetable broth, oregano, basil, and pepper.
5. Bring to a simmer and cook for 25-30 minutes until vegetables are tender.
6. Adjust seasoning if needed. Serve hot.

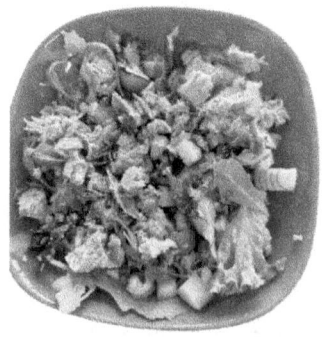

CONCLUSION

As you conclude this book specifically tailored for beginners like you, it's evident that knowledge is a powerful tool in managing this genetic kidney disorder.

I would like to believe that the journey through this book has equipped you with fundamental insights to help you navigate the complexities of PKD with confidence.

Starting with an understanding of the genetic underpinnings of PKD, the book elucidates the importance of early detection and monitoring.

By shedding light on the symptoms and risk factors, you are now equipped to recognize potential signs, facilitating timely intervention and improved outcomes.

The emphasis on lifestyle modifications and dietary considerations underscores the proactive role you can play in managing PKD.

Through accessible language and practical advice, the book has demystified the often-intricate realm of renal health, making it approachable for beginners like you.

Finally, the significance of regular medical check-ups and collaboration with healthcare professionals cannot be overstated. Do well to visit your health care provided or dietitian for professional advice.

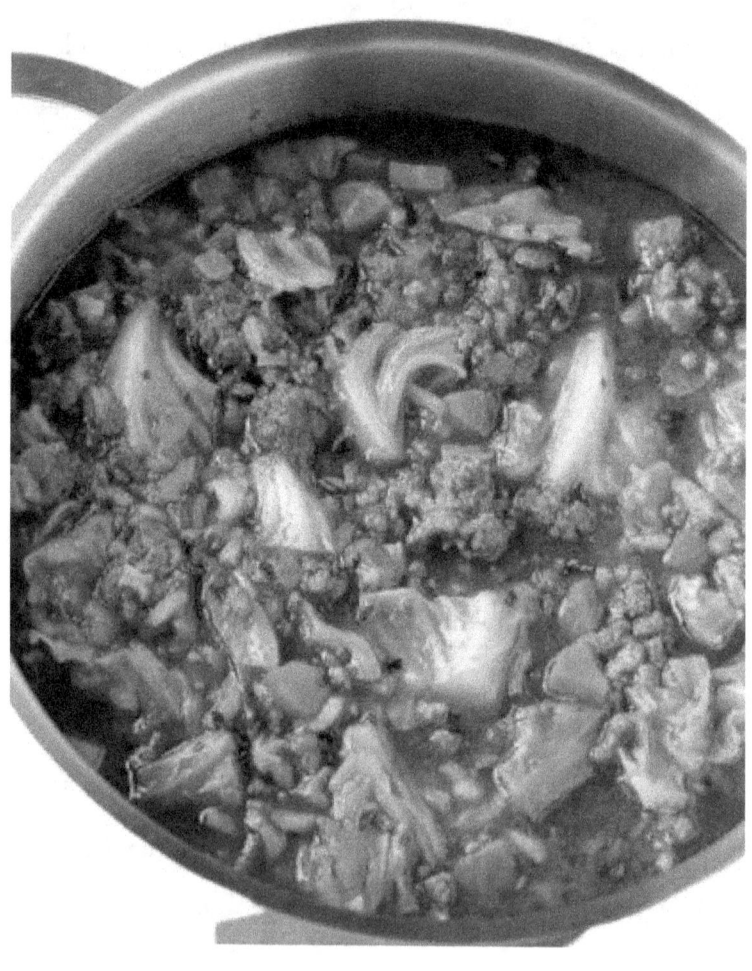